Homemade Deodorant

30 Organic Non-Toxic Deodorant and Body Spray Recipes to Keep You Dry And Smelling Fresh All Day Long!

Table of content

Introduction

I want to thank you and congratulate you for downloading the book "Homemade Deodorant: 30 Best Non-Toxic Organic Deodorant and Body Spray Recipes to Keep You Dry And Smelling Fresh All Day Long!"

This book contains proven steps and strategies on how to make your own deodorant, body sprays, and perfumes.

The fact is commercial deodorants are not what they used to be. They are full of chemicals, harmful additives, and dyes that have been proven to be carcinogens, meaning they can cause cancer. In addition, they are endocrine disruptors, so they make you more susceptible to hormone abnormalities, which can also lead to cancer.

The bottom line is that deodorant that you purchase from the store is not healthy for you, but you can make your own version that works just as well, and doesn't come with the added risk of breast cancer, liver disease, and many other terrible complications!

Find out how to make your own deodorant, body spray, and perfume throughout this book.

Chapter One – Why Use Organic Ingredients?

Deodorant is a habitual practice that just about no one actually thinks about. It's a convenient roll on liquid, spray or a traditional stick application. Its purpose is to make sure that when you lift up your arms, no one has the pleasant surprise of smelling something unpleasant. Deodorant is your defense against wet underarms and smelly armpits, but what's in the current deodorant you might be wearing?

In this chapter, we're going to go over some of the common ingredients found in the conventional deodorant you might be purchasing, and see if these odor and sweat blocking additives are what you really want stuck to your underarms all day.

Once you understand the ingredients in conventional deodorant, you'll know why you should use organic ingredients to make your own deodorant.

Aluminum

Aluminum is the main ingredient that's included in antiperspirant deodorants. This is a metal that's used to block your sweat glands, decreasing your capability to sweat by an average of twenty percent. The problem with this common metal is that it can cause serious health risks such as breast cancer and Alzheimer's disease.

Due to aluminum's main function being to block the sweat glands, what happens to all of your sweat? The underarms are closely linked to the lymph nodes, so this accumulation of toxins from your sweat not being perspired can potentially cause mayhem in your armpits. No amount of build-up of toxins in your body is good for you, and long-term build-up can cause cell mutation.

While the link between aluminum and breast cancer has controversial studies, it still convincing them with most breast cancer is developing in the upper outer quadrant of the breasts, which is the close a squadron to your armpit with lymph nodes are located, the long-term use of commercial deodorant with aluminum is factored into the formation of certain breast cancers.

In addition, women are more likely to shave under their arms, which mean excess aluminum is able to pass through this area more effectively. This could be the reason why breast cancer is more common amongst women.

Propylene Glycol

Another ingredient that's frequently used in deodorants is propylene glycol. Propylene glycol is a substance that is derived from petroleum and use to make a soft and silky consistency. It's a cheap ingredient that has a versatile function, and this is the reason it's so common in beauty products. Propylene glycol acts as a penetration enhancer, so if it's paired with harmful chemicals it will increase their absorption.

Recent studies have shown that propylene glycol is considered to be nontoxic to the body when it's ingested. It's eliminated from the body after a few hours, which is why it's considered nontoxic. However, there are reports of its potential toxicity being linked to issues such as:

* Cancer

* Developmental abnormalities

* Reproductive complications

* Endocrine complications

* Neurotoxicity

Propylene glycol has a single main concern beings that it's a skin sensitizer, which means it can cause allergic reactions such as irritant contact dermatitis, non-immunologic contact urticarial (hives), and allergic contact dermatitis.

Itching profusely under the arms can be very annoying, not to mention embarrassing.

Phthalates

This ingredient, also known as fragrance on the ingredient list, is a plasticizing chemical that's often used in many other beauty products due to their consistency and their capability to help dissolve some of the other ingredients.

The performance and the function of the ingredient seem to be more important to the conventional skin care brands than the quality and the safety of the ingredients.

This product helps your deodorant glide on smoothly, but what are the consequences of it being in your deodorant? It is worth having a temporary fix that could possibly cause a larger problem later on?

Phthalates are linked to many health issues and are considered endocrine disruptors. Once they are absorbed by your body, they act like estrogen, which not only conflict with hormonal function, but they also cause many other complications, such as:

- Decreased sperm count
- Infertility
- Prostate, breast, and ovarian cancer
- Lung, liver, and kidney damage
- Asthma
- Endometriosis
- Allergies

These are a probable human carcinogen and while the United States continues to regulate them, they're still very prevalent in many beauty products, including deodorants.

Sometimes, you might not consider the potential harm of a simple step of getting ready in the morning, but little do you know that your deodorant, antiperspirants, and your body sprays are all just another pitfall in an endless chemical burden of the conventional skin care products.

So skip the dangerous commercial deodorants, body sprays, perfumes, and mists, and try out some of the recipes in this book!

Chapter Two – Organic Deodorant Recipes

Homemade Deodorant with Shea Butter

Ingredients

- 3 Tbsp. Coconut Oil

- 2 Tbsp. Shea Butter

- 3 Tbsp. Baking Soda

- 2 Tbsp. Arrowroot Powder

- Essential Oils Of Your Choice

Directions

1. Melt the coconut oil and the Shea butter in a double boiler over medium heat until they're just melted. You want to combine in a quart sized glass mason jar with a lid instead and put this in a small saucepan of water until it's melted. This saves you a bowl and you can just designate this jar for this type of project and not need to wash it out. This can also be done in your microwave.

2. Remove this from the heat and add the arrowroot and the baking soda.

3. Mix it all together well.

4. Add the essential oils and then pour it all into a glass container to store it. It doesn't need to be refrigerated.

5. If you like, you can allow it to cool totally and put it into an old deodorant stick for easier usage, thought it could melt in the summer.

Take note this recipe can take a few hours to completely harden and the process can be sped up by putting it in the refrigerator for a few minutes.

Coconut Oil Homemade Deodorant Recipe

Ingredients

- 6 Tbsp. Coconut Oil
- ¼ C. Baking Soda
- ¼ C. Arrowroot Powder
- Essential Oils Of Your Choice

Directions

1. Mix the arrowroot powder and the baking soda together in a medium bowl.

2. Mash the oil with a fork until it's well incorporated.

3. Add the oils if you prefer them.

4. Store it in a small, glass jar or an old deodorant container.

Deodorant Bar Recipe

Ingredients

- ½ C. Coconut Oil

- ½ C. Shea Butter

- ½ C. Beeswax

- 1 Tsp. Vitamin E Oil

- 3 Tbsp. Baking Soda

- ½ C. Organic Arrowroot Powder

- 3 Capsules High Quality Probiotics

- 20 Drops Essential Oil Of Your Choice

Directions

1. Combine the coconut oil, shea butter and the beeswax in a double boiler or a glass bowl that's set over a smaller saucepan with an inch of water in it. You can also use a quart sized glass mason jar with a lid and put it in a small saucepan of hot water. This saves you the bowl and you can designate the jar for this type of project and not have to wash it out.

2. Turn the burner on and bring your water to a boil. Stir the ingredients continuously until they're melted and smooth.

3. Remove them from the heat and add the vitamin E oil, arrowroot powder, baking soda, probiotics, and the essential oils. Be sure the oil isn't too hot

so the heat won't kill your probiotics. If you can touch it without being burnt, it's not too hot.

4. Gently stir it until all the ingredients are well combined.

5. If you want to make this into bars, then pour it into muffin tins or another mold that will hold liquid. If you are going to put it into an old deodorant container and use it like stick deodorant, then let the mix harden for around twenty minutes. When it's around the consistency of peanut butter, use a spoon to scoop it into the tube and pack it down in. Then, allow the cup to stay off overnight to completely harden the deodorant before using it.

Homemade Deodorant for Sensitive Skin

Ingredients

- ¾ C. Cornstarch or Arrowroot Powder
- ¼ C. Baking Soda
- 6 Tbsp. Melted Coconut Oil

Directions

1. Combine the arrowroot powder or cornstarch with the baking soda.

2. Add four tablespoons of the coconut oil to the mix and mash it down with a fork until it's well combined. Keep adding the coconut oil until the deodorant reaches a consistency you like.

3. Transfer the mix to a jar that has a tight fitting lid.

4. To use the deodorant, apply a little under your arms with your fingertips as it's needed.

Homemade Deodorant Recipe for Sensitive Skin

Ingredients

- ¾ C. Cornstarch or Arrowroot Powder
- ¼ C. Diatomaceous Earth (Food Grade)
- 9 Tbsp. Melted Coconut Oil

Directions

1. Combine the arrowroot or cornstarch with the diatomaceous earth.

2. Add six tablespoons of melted oil and mix it up with a fork. Keep adding the oil until the deodorant has reached your desired consistency.

3. Then transfer to a jar that has a tight fitting lid and apply a small amount under your arms when it's needed.

All-Natural Homemade Deodorant Recipe

Ingredients

- ½ Tbsp. Baking Soda

- ⅛ C. Arrowroot Powder

- ⅛ C. Cocoa Butter

- ⅛ C. Shea Butter

- 5 Vitamin E Oil Drops

- 25-40 Drops Your Chosen Essential Oil

Directions

1. Using a Pyrex measuring glass, combine the shea butter and the cocoa butter.

2. Use a double boiler to heat the oils over medium heat until they are melted.

3. Remove them from the heat and stir in the baking soda and the arrowroot powder.

4. Stir in the vitamin E oil and your essential oils.

5. Carefully pour this mix into two ounce tins, filling them to the top, but making sure not to spill it over.

6. Put the lids on the container but don't press down to lock them. Just allow them to rest on the top to help prevent any dust from settling into the deodorant as it settles.

7. Let it completely cool and solidify, which can take six or more hours. Letting it sit overnight is best.

Homemade Deodorant

Ingredients

- ½ C. Coconut Oil

- ½ C. Baking Soda

- 40-60 Essential Oil Drops

- Empty Deodorant Container

Directions

1. Put the oil into a bowl.

2. Mix the baking soda into it.

3. Add the essential oil and mix well.

4. Store it in your deodorant container or in a glass jar.

Recipe for Homemade Summer Deodorant

Ingredients

- ¼ C. Cornstarch

- ¼ C. Baking Soda

- 3 Tbsp. coconut Oil

- 1 Tbsp. Beeswax, Grated
- 5 Tea Tree Oil Drops
- 5 Essential Oil Drops of Your choice

Directions

1. Start by melting the oil and the wax together in a double boiler. Rest a heat-proof bowl inside a saucepan that has an inch worth of water in the bottom. Heat it gently, stirring continuously, until the wax has melted.

2. Add the rest of the ingredients.

3. Stir it together. At this point, you will have a runny paste or slurry. This changes quickly.

4. Work quickly by pouring the paste into the empty deodorant container. By the end of this step, you might have to scrape the last bit of paste into the container and push it down, smoothing the top. That's how quickly it will begin to solidify.

Lemon Juice

Ingredients

- Lemon Juice

Directions

1. Many people like to use lemon as a natural deodorizer. Lemon juice contains citric acid that helps kill the odor-causing bacteria under your arms. Use a lemon slice on your armpits every morning. Remember, don't use lemon juice on any recently shaved areas, though!

Rubbing Alcohol

Ingredients

- Rubbing Alcohol
- Cotton Ball

Directions

1. Rubbing alcohol is another way to kill odor causing bacteria. It's inexpensive and very easy to use, too. You can just fill a spray bottle with rubbing alcohol and spritz it under your arms, or you can use a cotton ball and gently dab it on. Adding an essential oil will make it into a pretty, scented spritzer, too.

Detoxifying Deodorant

Ingredients

- 5 Tbsp. Coconut Oil
- 3 Tbsp. Baking Soda

- 3 Tbsp. Arrowroot Powder

- 2 Tbsp. Bentonite Clay

- 20 Tea Tree Oil Drops

Directions

1. Put everything in a mixing bowl in the order that it's listed in. because coconut oil is a solid when it's at room temperature, it has to be heated to be able to mix it easily. With your clean hands, knead the mixture until everything makes a smooth paste. Then transfer this paste to a glass jar or a deodorant stick.

2. The paste will thicken after you let it cool at room temperature. To apply it, just rub your finger on the top of the paste and scoop out a little amount to rub on your underarms. The pate will melt right into the sick and absorb quickly.

All-Natural Coconut Deodorant

Ingredients

- ¼ C. Coconut Oil

- ⅛ C. Cornstarch

- ⅛ C. Arrowroot Powder

- Essential Oils of Your Choice

- 1 Tbsp. Baking Soda

Directions

1. Combine the oil, cornstarch, baking soda, and the arrowroot powder in a mixing bowl. When it's well combined, add in your essential oil a few drops at a time until you get to the scent you prefer.

2. Pour it into an empty deodorant container or just pour it into a small mason jar and refrigerator it for fifteen minutes. Remove it from the refrigerator and use it as you need it.

3. If you're using a mason jar, you'll need to chip out some little piece and then rub it onto your armpit. The deodorant melts and applies smoothly to your skin.

DIY Natural Deodorant Solid Recipe

Ingredients

- 2 Tbsp. Coconut Oil
- 1 Tbsp. Beeswax
- 1 Tbsp. Shea Butter
- 2 Tbsp. Arrowroot Powder
- 1 ½ Tbsp. Bentonite Clay
- 1 Tbsp. Baking Soda
- 2 Drops Citronella Essential Oil

- 2 Drops Lemongrass Essential Oil

- 2 Drops Tea Tree Essential Oil

Directions

1. In a double boiler, add the shea butter, coconut oil, and the wax. Bring it all to a boil over medium heat and stir until the wax and oils are melted.

2. Remove it from the heat and add in the bentonite clay, baking soda, arrowroot powder, and the essential oils. Mix it all well.

3. Pour the liquid into some silicone muffin molds or a five ounce container, such as an empty deodorant container.

4. Let it cool down and solidify for around two to three hours. The wax will help keep it solid so you can use it as a traditional deodorant.

Easy Deodorant

Ingredients

- ¼ C. Baking Soda

- ¼ C. Cornstarch or Arrowroot Powder

- 5 Tbsp. Coconut Oil

Directions

1. Combine the arrowroot powder and the baking soda together with a fork. Start with around four tablespoons of the oil and then add it to the baking soda mix. Work it into a paste.

2. Add the rest if you feel you need to.

3. You can store this in a small container or put it in an empty deodorant stick.

Vitamin E Deodorant

Ingredients

- 3 Tbsp. Shea Butter

- 2 Tbsp. Cornstarch

- 3 Tbsp. Baking Soda

- 2 Tbsp. Cocoa Butter

- 2 Vitamin E Caps

- Essential Oil of your choice

Directions

1. Melt everything but the oil together and stir it.

2. The mix in the oil and pour it into a container, and put the container in the refrigerator to let it set.

3. This recipe will fill a ¼ pint jar.

Chapter Three – Organic Body Spray Recipes

Vanilla and Ylang-Ylang Body Spray

Ingredients

- 18 Vanilla Oleoresin Drops
- 2 Ylang-Ylang Drops
- ¼ C. Witch Hazel with Alcohol

Directions

1. Mix everything together in a dark colored spray bottle and store it in a dark place.

Vanilla and Sweet Orange Body Spray

Ingredients

- 16 Vanilla Oleoresin Drops
- 4 Sweet Orange Essential Oil Drops
- ¼ C. Witch Hazel with Alcohol

Directions

1. Mix everything together in a dark colored bottle and store it in a dark place.

Vanilla and Coffee Body Spray

- 16 Vanilla Oleoresin Drops
- 4 Coffee Essential Oil Drops
- ¼ C. Witch Hazel with Alcohol

Directions

1. Mix everything together in a dark colored spray bottle and store it in a dark, cool place.

Vanilla Clove Body Oil Spray

Ingredients

- ¼ C. Almond Oil
- ½ tsp. Vanilla Extract or Essential Oil
- 3 Drops Clove Oil
- Spray Bottle

Directions

1. Combine the ingredients and pour it into a small spray bottle.

Orange Blossom Body Spray

Ingredients

- 1 oz. Filtered Water
- 90 Drops Orange Essential Oil
- ½ tsp. Vegetable Glycerine

Directions

1. Add everything to a small spray bottle, shake to combine and spritz onto your skin. Be sure to rub it in.

Bohemian Patchouli Body Spray

Ingredients

- 1 oz. filtered water
- ⅛ tsp. Tunisian Patchouli Essential Oil

- ½ tsp. Vegetable Glycerine

Directions

1. Mix it together in a small, glass spray bottle and shake it well. Shake it before you use it.

Citrus Energy Natural Body Spray

Ingredients

- 1 oz. Distilled Water
- ½ oz. Witch Hazel with Alcohol
- ½ oz. Vegetable Glycerin
- 10 Grapefruit Essential Oil Drops
- 4 Lime Essential Oil Drops
- 4 Lemon Essential Oil Drops

Directions

1. Mix everything together in a small glass bottle and shake it well. Shake it before every use.

Orange Vanilla Natural Body Spray

Ingredients

- 1 oz. Distilled Water
- ½ oz. Witch Hazel with Alcohol
- ½ oz. Vegetable Glycerin
- ⅛ tsp. Vanilla Extract
- 10 Drops Orange Essential Oil

Directions

1. Mix it all together in a small glass bottle and shake it well. Shake it before every use.

Purifying Linen and Body Spray

Ingredients

- 1 C. Water
- 120 Drops Essential Oil
    - 20 Drops Peppermint
    - 40 Drops Lemon
    - 40 Drops Eucalyptus
- Dark Brown Spray Bottle (Glass)

Directions

1. Pour the water into the bottle

2. Add the essential oils.

3. Shake before you use it.

Moisturizing Body Spray

Ingredients

- ¼ C. Distilled Water

- 1 ½ tsp. Vegetable Glycerin

- 1 tsp. Grapeseed Oil

- 5 Drops Vitamin E Oil

- 10 Drops Essential Oil

Directions

1. Combine all the ingredients and carefully pour them into a small spray bottle, around three ounces. Shake it well before you use it.

2. Spray it liberally on your body as it's needed, especially after you shower. Rub it into your skin.

Lemon, Lavender, and Vanilla Body Spray

Ingredients

- 1 Glass Spray Bottle, 4 oz.

- 3 ½ oz. Vodka

- 5 Drops Lemon essential Oil

- 15 Drops Lavender Essential Oil

- 30 Drops Vanilla Essential Oil

Directions

1. Combine everything into a spray bottle and shake it well before using it.

Woodland Body Spray

Ingredients

- 4 Drops Spruce Essential Oil

- 2 Drops Cedarwood Essential Oil

- 2 Drops Fir Needle Essential Oil

- 1 Drop Bergamot Essential Oil

- 1 Drop Vetiver Essential Oil

- 1 tsp. Jojoba Oil

Directions

1. Add all the essential oils into the glass bottle and mix the oils with a wooden skewer or by shaking it gently.

2. Add the oil and shake it again.

3. Add more essential oil if you want it to be a little stronger.

Cucumber, Aloe Body Mist

Ingredients

- 1 Squeeze Lemon

- 1 Cucumber

- 1 tsp. Aloe Vera Gel

- 1 Tbsp. Rosewater

Directions

1. Peel the cucumber and dice it into pieces. Put them in a blender and pulse it on high for around a minute.

2. Cover a bowl with some cheese cloth and then strain the juice into the bowl.

3. Add the rest of the ingredients to the bowl and mix it thoroughly.

4. Transfer the mix to a spray bottle and you're done. You can add a little distilled water if you feel you need to dilute it a bit.

5. Store it in the refrigerator so it doesn't spoil. It'll last around a week.

Tropical Body Mist

Ingredients

- 1 oz. Distilled Water

- 10ml Rose Hydrosol

- 2 tsp. Vanilla Extract

- 1 tsp. Vodka

- 1 Tbsp. Vegetable Glycerin

- 1 Tbsp. Coconut Oil

- 5 Grapefruit Essential Oil drops

- 15 Neroli Essential Oil Drops

Directions

1. Begin by filling the spray bottle with some lukewarm distilled water and the hydrosol.

2. Add the vegetable glycerin slowly and then add the coconut oil. Use a wooden skewer to mix the two.

3. Make sure you're happy with the scent thus far and the consistency.

4. Then add the essential oils and close the spray bottle. Shake it well.

5. Let it rest a few hours before you use it the first time.

6. Always shake it well to make sure all the ingredients are mixed well.

Vanilla Cardamom Mist

Ingredients

- 6 Cardamom Seeds
- ½ C. Water
- 1 tsp. Vanilla Extract

Directions

1. Crack the seeds to expose their pods.

2. Put the bits of cardamom into a saucepan with the water and bring it to a boil. Remove it from the heat.

3. Let the cardamom water cool totally.

4. Transfer the scented water to a spray bottle.

5. Add the vanilla, seal the spray bottle, and shake it.

6. Adjust the amount of vanilla extract to your preference and store in a cool, dry place.

Grapefruit Mist

Ingredients

- 10 Drops Grapefruit Essential Oil
- Vodka
- Distilled Water
- Glass Spray Bottle

Directions

1. Fill the glass bottle up around two-thirds of the way with the vodka and add a few drops of the essential oil before you fill the bottle up the rest of the way with the distilled water.

Chapter Four – Organic Perfume Recipes

Solid Perfume

Ingredients

- 1 ½ Tbsp. Beeswax
- 1 ½ Tbsp. Olive Oil
- 40 Drops Essential Oil of your choice

Directions

1. Fill up a pan with half a cup of water and put it on the burner. Turn the burner heat to medium. Put the wax beads into a heatproof glass bowl and put it inside the pan. When it's melted, mix in the oil. Let it melt for another five minutes.

2. Remove the glass owl from the pan and quickly stir in the essential oil. Pour this into its final container.

3. The essential oils will smell strong in the beginning, but they will fade over time.

4. To use the solid perfume, wipe it on the interior of your wrist for a clean scent that'll last all day.

California Citrus Sunshine

Ingredients

- 1 Tbsp. Jojoba Oil

- 2 Tbsp. Grain Alcohol

- 7 Drops Sweet Orange Essential Oil

- 7 Drops Grapefruit Essential Oil

- 7 Drops Peppermint Essential Oil

- 7 Drops Lavender Essential Oil

- 1 Tbsp. Distilled Water

Directions

1. Begin by adding the jojoba to a glass container and then add the alcohol. It's important to use glass and not plastic.

2. Add the essential oils in the order they were listed in on the ingredients list.

3. Add the distilled water using a dropper.

4. Mix the ingredient well and transfer them to a dark container for forty-eight hours up to six weeks. The longer it sits, the stronger the scent is going to be.

5. Transfer it to a pretty perfume bottle after it's reached your desired scent.

Solid Shimmer Perfume

Ingredients

- 2 tsp. almond oil
- Essential oils of your choice
- 1 oz. beeswax

Directions

1. To make the solid perfume, combine the almond oil with the essential oils until you reach your desired scent.

2. The melt the wax and in a small glass in your microwave and add the oil mix. Stir it to combine it. Then pour it into a small mold to let it harden.

3. Add a small amount of shimmery eye shadow to give it some sparkle.

How to make Solid Essential Oil Perfume

Ingredients

- 1 Tbsp. beeswax
- 1 ½ Tbsp. Jojoba Oil
- 70 Drops Essential Oil

Directions

1. Grate or chop the beeswax finely and put it in the milk jug. Measure the oil into a small glass and then add the essential oil drops to your desired scent.

2. Melt the wax by filling the saucepan with about an inch of water, and then putting a glass container in the water. Put the beeswax into the glass and avoid spilling any water into the glass. Bring the water to a simmer and melt the wax.

3. As soon as it's done, add the oil and stir it with a wooden skewer until it's well combined. Carefully remove it from the hot water. The glass is going to be hot, so use a cloth to protect your hands.

4. Quickly pour the wax into containers and let it rest for half an hour or until it's cooled down. To use it, just rub the wax surface with your fingertips and then rub it on your wrists and neck.

Lavender Vanilla Mist

Ingredients

- ½ C. Vodka

- 2 Tbsp. Vegetable Glycerin

- 1 C. Dried Lavender Flowers

- 2 Vanilla Beans

- 10 Drops Vanilla Extract

- 15 Drops lavender Essential Oil

Directions

1. Slice the vanilla bean open with a sharp knife.

2. Put the beans and the flowers in a large glass jar with a lid.

3. Pour the vodka into the jar and secure the lid.

4. Let the mix infuse for a week.

5. Strain and discard your vanilla beans and your lavender flowers.

6. Add the lavender essential oil, the glycerin, and the vanilla extract to the reserved liquids and stir it well.

7. Replace the lid and let it age for four to six weeks.

8. Strain the perfume once again through a paper filter and then transfer it to a decorate spray bottle.

Midnight Perfume

Ingredients

- 2 Tbsp. Jojoba Oil or Grape Seed Oil

- 6 Tbsp. Vodka

- 2 ½ Tbsp. Distilled Spring Water

- Funnel

- Coffee Filter

- Essential Oils

  - 15 Drops Clove Oil

  - 6 Drops Cedarwood Oil

  - 9 Drops lavender Oil

- 2 Dark Colored Glass Bottles

- Decorate Perfume Bottle

Directions

1. Start by cleaning the bottles, either in the dishwasher on the hottest setting or with some hot, soapy water. Put the bottles on a rimmed baking sheet and dry them in an oven set at 230 degrees Fahrenheit. Remove them from the oven when they're totally dry.

2. Put a lid on one of them and set it aside until you need it, which will anywhere from two days to six weeks later.

3. Put the carrier oil in one of your bottles.

4. Then add the essential oils.

5. Add the vodka.

6. Put the lid on top of the bottle and shake it well for several minutes.

7. Let it rest for forty-eight hours to six weeks.

8. The scent changes over time, becoming its strongest around six weeks.

9. Check it weekly and once you're happy with the scent, add two tablespoons of spring water to it and shake it well for a minute.

10. Put the coffee filter into the funnel and transfer your perfume from the bottle it's in to the perfume bottle. Label it and store it in a cool, dark place.

Citrus Lavender

Ingredients

- 2 tsp. Beeswax
- 48 Drops Essential Oils
    - 12 Drops Sweet Orange Essential Oil
    - 12 Drops Lemon Essential Oil
    - 12 Drops lavender Essential Oil
    - 12 Drops Bergamot Essential Oil
- 2 tsp. Jojoba Oil
- ½ oz. Tin

Directions

1. It's a good idea to blend the oils first before you begin working with the beeswax because it will harden very quickly.

2. Put all your essential oils into one cup so you can pour them into the beeswax mix when it's time.

3. You can play around with the amount of oil that you use and try to substitute different ones if you don't like the ones that were listed.

4. You can also use sweet almond oil for the carrier oil, too.

5. In another cup from the essential oils, measure out two teaspoons of the oil of your choice.

6. Measuring out the oil ahead of time saves you from having to rush around once the wax has melted.

7. If you have pellets of wax, then measure out two teaspoons of them into a small saucepan over medium to low heat.

8. If you have a block of wax, then you should grate off around a tablespoon of wax and then melt them in the pot. Then measure to make sure you have two teaspoons.

9. After you measure, you may find you have to heat the wax up again in the pan a few more seconds because it might begin to harden after you pour it into a measuring spoon.

10. Once you have the two teaspoons of the melted beeswax, add the carrier oil to it and stir it around until they're both combined.

11. Then take the pot off the burner and very quickly add the essential oils. Stir until they are well combined.

12. As quickly as you can, pour the mix into the container.

13. Cover it and allow it to rest ten minutes before you enjoy it.

Conclusion

Thank you again for downloading this book!

I hope this book was able to help you to learn how to make your own deodorant.

The next step is to gather up your ingredients and start cooking!

Finally, if you enjoyed this book, please take the time to share your thoughts and post a review on Amazon. It'd be greatly appreciated!

Thank you and good luck!

FREE Bonus Reminder

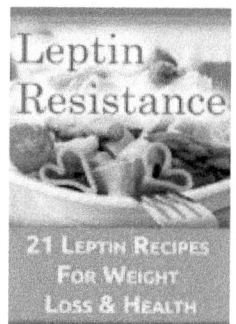

If you have not grabbed it yet, please go ahead and download your special bonus report *"Leptin Resistance. 21 Leptin Recipes For Weight Loss & Healthy Living"*.

Simply Click the Button Below

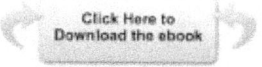

OR **Go to This Page**

http://easyweightlossway.com/free/

BONUS #2: More Free & Discounted Books

Do you want to receive more Free & Discounted Books?

We have a mailing list where we send out our new Books when they go free or with a discount on Kindle. Click on the link below to sign up for Free & Discount Book Promotions.

=> Sign Up for Free & Discount Book Promotions <=

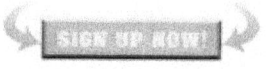

OR Go to this URL

www.ingramcontent.com/pod-product-compliance
Lightning Source LLC
Chambersburg PA
CBHW072020290526

45787CB00013B/1414